THE PERFECT COLLAGEN DIET COOKBOOK

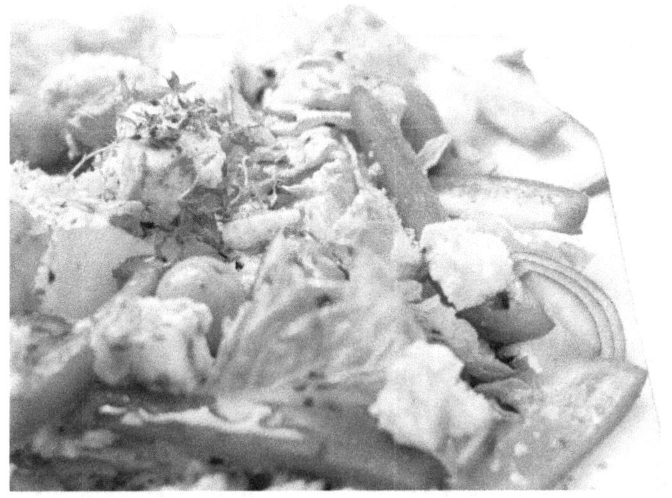

Revitalize Your Radiance with Delicious Recipes for Vibrant Skin, Hair, and Joints

Isabelle Hartley

OTHER BOOKS BY THIS AUTHOR

1. GASTROPARESIS DIET RECIPES COOKBOOK
2. HIGH CALORIES DIET COOKBOOK
3. DIET FOR WOMEN OVER FORTY
4. HASHIMOTO RECIPES COOKBOOK
5. JUICING RECIPES FOR CANCER
6. IVF DIET COOKBOOK FOR BEGINNERS
7. LOW SUGAR DIET GUIDE FOR BEGINNERS
8. RAW FOODS RECIPES COOKBOOK
9. SMOOTHIES RECIPES FOR ANTI-INFLAMMATION
10. MEDITERRANEAN DIET FOR PREGNANT WOMEN

TABLE OF CONTENTS

Introduction

I'd like to begin this book with a tale of Samuel. Samuel, who was 75 years old, was suffering from a disorder connected to collagen that was causing his skin to become less elastic and his joints to become stiff. In an attempt to restore his vigor, he set out to find the ideal diet for collagen.

And then Samuel's days became an adventure in food, the smell of bone broth filling his kitchen. With the help of a frayed cookbook, he painstakingly prepared dishes brimming with collagen-building components. Vibrant veggies, lean meats, and a hint of exotic spices that promised internal healing were all part of his regimen.

Months passed into weeks, and Samuel's change was evident. His once painful joints moved with unexpected ease, and his aged skin had a refreshed sheen when he looked in the mirror. The populace was in awe of the elderly man's amazing transformation—he appeared to have rolled back the years.

As word of Samuel's adventure spread, the neighborhood became interested. Before long, talk of the "Perfect Collagen Diet" that had come to be associated with Samuel's health was rife throughout the area. He was sought after for advice by friends and neighbors, and the cookbook that had been his constant companion turned into a treasured possession for people on a similar path to well-being.

Once a symbol of the difficulties associated with growing older, Samuel was now an inspiration. His narrative struck a chord with those struggling with ailments linked to collagen even outside the boundaries of his tiny community. Samuel's "Perfect Collagen Diet Cookbook" was a ray of hope that helped a great number of people live better, more energetic lives.

During his elderly years, Samuel shared his story with those who were looking for comfort in the cookbook, which gave him a sense of purpose in addition to improved health.

CHAPTER 1

Welcome to the world of the Collagen Diet, a revolutionary dietary strategy that uses collagen's potential to improve well-being. Our skin, joints, and connective tissues require collagen, the most abundant protein in our body, to be structurally intact. But aging, stress, and eating poorly may all lower our collagen levels, which can cause a host of problems.

The foundation of the Collagen Condition Diet is centered on using carefully chosen meals to promote and restore the body's synthesis of collagen. Whole, nutrient-dense meals high in amino acids, vitamins, and minerals—building blocks of collagen—are the focus of this diet. Collagen-rich bone broths, lean meats, colorful veggies, and fruits with pro-collagen qualities are essential ingredients.

Starting this journey has several advantages, including boosting intestinal health, improving muscle tone, and encouraging skin elasticity and joint flexibility. The Collagen Condition meal is a comprehensive strategy for nourishing your body from the inside out, not simply a meal plan. You may experience the possibility of better digestion, glowing skin, and a resurgence of energy as you go through the tasty and nutritious meals in this meal plan.

The Collagen Condition Diet encourages you to go on a journey of holistic nourishment and culinary inquiry, regardless of whether you're looking to treat particular collagen-related issues or are interested in making a proactive investment in your general health. Become one of the innumerable people who have already reaped the benefits of eating foods high in collagen and unleash a younger, healthier you.

THE COLLAGEN DISORDER

A variety of illnesses that impact the body's capacity to create, use, or preserve collagen—a vital protein that gives different tissues shape and support—are referred to as collagen diseases. Investigating the many kinds, origins, and manifestations of abnormalities in collagen metabolism is necessary to comprehend these disorders.

Types of Collagen Conditions:

1. The collection of hereditary illnesses known as the Ehlers-Danlos Syndromes (EDS) affects the production of collagen.

There are several subgroups with unique clinical characteristics, such as skin fragility, joint hypermobility, and hypermobility.

EDS affects several body systems and can range in severity from moderate to severe.

2. Osteogenesis Imperfecta (OI): Also referred to as "brittle bone disease," OI is caused by genetic abnormalities that impact collagen, namely Type I collagen.

characterized by brittle bones, skeletal abnormalities, and fracture vulnerability.

3. Rheumatoid arthritis (RA): An autoimmune disease that causes inflammation in the joints by attacking the synovium, a collagen-rich tissue.

Joint abnormalities can arise from chronic inflammation causing damage to collagen.

4. Systemic Lupus Erythematosus (SLE): This autoimmune disease causes the immune system to attack different tissues, such as the skin, joints, and organs that are high in collagen.

Common symptoms include organ inflammation, joint discomfort, and skin rashes.

5. Scleroderma: This condition causes aberrant collagen synthesis, which thickens and fibroses the skin.

6. May have an impact on internal organs, leading to respiratory, gastrointestinal, and cardiovascular system issues.

Causes of Collagen Disorders:

1. Genetic Mutations: A number of disorders involving collagen, including Osteogenesis

Imperfecta and Ehlers-Danlos Syndromes, have a genetic foundation.

Collagen synthesis and structure can be disturbed by inherited mutations.

2. Autoimmune Responses: Diseases such as Systemic Lupus Erythematosus and Rheumatoid Arthritis are caused by the immune system mistakenly attacking tissues that are high in collagen.

This immunological reaction leads to tissue damage and chronic inflammation.

3. Environmental Factors: Toxin exposure from the environment, UV rays, and certain drugs may hasten the deterioration of collagen.

Lifestyle decisions like smoking and eating poorly can also affect the health of your collagen.

4. Aging: The quantity and quality of collagen decrease as we age naturally.

Declining skin suppleness, stiff joints, and wrinkles are all caused by less collagen.

5. Infections and Prolonged Inflammation: These conditions might hinder the production of collagen and encourage its deterioration.

For example, scleroderma causes inflammation that causes an overabundance of collagen to form.

Symptoms
1. Joint stiffness and pain are common in diseases like rheumatoid arthritis and some Ehlers-Danlos syndrome subtypes. Collagen deterioration in the joints causes pain and limited movement.
2. Skin Abnormalities: Skin-related symptoms are a common manifestation of Ehlers-Danlos syndromes and Scleroderma.
3. Hyperelasticity, bruising easily, or, on the other hand, skin tightening and thickening are a few examples of these.

4. Bone Fragility: The hallmark of Osteogenesis Imperfecta is brittle, fracture-prone bones.

5. The strength of collagen in bone tissue is compromised by genetic abnormalities.

6. Hypermobility: Weakening collagen causes joint hypermobility in some Ehlers-Danlos syndrome types.

7. Instability and joint dislocations can result from excessive joint flexibility.

8. Organ Involvement: Internal organs may be impacted by collagen disorders such as Scleroderma.

9. Lung fibrosis, heart problems, and trouble swallowing are just a few of the symptoms.

10. weariness: The body's attempts to heal tissues rich in collagen and chronic inflammation can both lead to weariness. People who have autoimmune collagen disorders frequently feel exhausted all the time.

Identification and Handling:
Clinical Evaluation: A comprehensive clinical examination by medical specialists is frequently necessary for the diagnosis of collagen disorders.

To find particular mutations linked to hereditary collagen diseases, genetic testing may be used.

Ultrasounds, MRIs, and X-rays can all be used to evaluate the health of your bones and joints, particularly if you have musculoskeletal issues.

Blood Tests: Blood tests that identify certain antibodies are frequently used to diagnose autoimmune collagen disorders.

Inflammatory markers might also be evaluated.
Skin Biopsy: A biopsy may be carried out to look under a microscope at collagen in circumstances where skin involvement is suspected.

This can help in the diagnosis of diseases such as Scleroderma.

Depending on the severity of the particular collagen issue, different treatments are used.

A treatment approach frequently includes physical therapy, medications, and lifestyle changes.

While studies on collagen supplementation's effectiveness are still being conducted, some people see it as a management strategy.

It's generally advised to eat a diet high in elements that promote collagen formation.

The management of pain linked with collagen problems often involves medication, physical therapy, and lifestyle modifications.

The goal of pain management techniques is to enhance the lives of those who suffer from these ailments.

The complexity of diseases linked to collagen is being uncovered by ongoing study, providing fresh perspectives on possible therapeutic approaches. Prospective treatments might benefit from developments in precision medicine, genetic medicines, and a better comprehension of the immune system's involvement in collagen disorders.

To sum up, problems related to collagen comprise a wide variety of illnesses that have different autoimmune, genetic, and environmental causes. Comprehending the many kinds, origins, and manifestations is essential for precise identification and efficient handling. The goal is to improve the lives of those impacted by abnormalities in collagen metabolism by developing tailored medicines that target the underlying processes of these illnesses as medical research advances.

CHAPTER 2

FOODS TO EAT OR AVOID

A Collagen Condition Diet is centered around consuming foods that promote collagen synthesis, support connective tissue health, and reduce inflammation. Equally important is avoiding foods that may contribute to collagen degradation or exacerbate inflammation. Here's a comprehensive guide to the foods to include and those to steer clear of on a Collagen Condition Diet:

Foods to Include:

Bone broth: Packed in proline and glycine, two amino acids essential to the synthesis of collagen.

provide minerals that promote the general health of the bones and joints.

Lean Proteins: Lean beef cuts, fish, poultry, and turkey are all great sources of high-quality protein.

Tissue healing and collagen formation depend on protein.

Bright Vegetables: Antioxidants from bell peppers, carrots, spinach, and sweet potatoes help fight oxidative stress.

Antioxidants aid in preventing collagen deterioration.

Berries: Antioxidants and vitamin C are abundant in blueberries, strawberries, and raspberries.

Vitamin C keeps skin supple and is essential for the creation of collagen.

Citrus Fruits: Vitamin C is found in oranges, lemons, and grapefruits, and it helps to produce collagen.

Another antioxidant that guards against damage from free radicals is vitamin C.

Nuts and Seeds: Zinc and omega-3 fatty acids may be found in almonds, walnuts, chia seeds, and flaxseeds.

Collagen production and skin health are enhanced by zinc and omega-3 fatty acids.

Fish: Omega-3 fatty acids are abundant in fatty fish, such as mackerel and salmon.

Omega-3 fatty acids promote healthy skin and lessen inflammation.

Avocado: Rich in wholesome fats that promote collagen production and nurture the skin.

Packed with antioxidant vitamin E, which guards against oxidative stress.

Leafy Greens: Rich in vitamins A and C include kale, spinach, and Swiss chard.

These vitamins are necessary for healthy skin and the synthesis of collagen.

Foods High in Probiotics: Fermented foods like sauerkraut, kefir, and yogurt all improve gut health.

Decreased inflammation is associated with a healthy gut flora.

Foods to Avoid:
Processed Sugar: Consuming a lot of sugar can cause glycation, which deteriorates collagen and hastens the aging process.

Steer clear of sugary drinks, sweets, and snacks.

Processed meals: A lot of chemicals and preservatives found in highly processed meals can aggravate inflammation.

When possible, choose entire, unprocessed meals.

Drinking too much alcohol can cause the skin to become dehydrated and disrupt the production of collagen.

Drink less alcohol and drink plenty of water to keep hydrated.

Highly Processed Meats: Preservatives and chemicals connected to inflammation may be present in some processed meats.

Select lean, fresh meats over processed ones.

Trans Fats: Prone to inflammation, trans fats are included in a lot of fried and processed meals.

Examine food labels and steer clear of trans fat-containing items.

Overdosing on Caffeine: Although a modest amount of caffeine is usually safe, too much of it can cause the skin to become dehydrated.

Consume enough water in addition to a moderate amount of coffee.

High-Sodium Foods: Consuming too much salt can cause water retention, which can change the look of skin.

Limit processed meals rich in salt.

Gluten (if intolerant): Inflammation may be exacerbated in certain people with collagen-related disorders due to gluten sensitivity.

Try gluten-free options if you're intolerant.

Dairy (if intolerant): Some people may get inflammatory when they consume dairy.

If dairy bothers you, go for lactose-free or alternative dairy products.

Artificial Additives: Processed foods include preservatives and additives that may aggravate inflammation.

Examine product labels and select whole-food, natural choices.

Adopting a Collagen Condition Diet entails making deliberate decisions to promote the health of collagen and general wellbeing. Give priority to eating complete, nutrient-dense foods that are packed with important minerals, vitamins, and antioxidants. A comprehensive strategy for controlling collagen issues can also include eating a diverse and balanced diet, staying hydrated, and taking into account any food sensitivities that each individual may have. Always seek the advice of a trained dietitian or healthcare provider for individualized dietary recommendations based on individual health requirements.

CHAPTER 3

BENEFITS OF ADOPTING A COLLAGEN DIET

Adopting a diet high in collagen has several advantages for your health beyond your skin. The most prevalent protein in the body, collagen, is essential for preserving the structural integrity of a variety of tissues. A collagen diet has been shown to have a good effect on several elements of health and well-being.

1. Better Skin Health: Increased Elasticity: Collagen gives the skin structural support, which helps to maintain its firmness and suppleness. Fine lines and wrinkles appear less when a diet high in collagen promotes the synthesis of new collagen.

Hydration: Collagen keeps the skin hydrated, avoiding dryness and encouraging a smooth complexion. Maintaining a healthy skin barrier through enough hydration lowers the likelihood of irritation and inflammation.

2. Bone and Joint Support: Cartilage Preservation: A significant portion of cartilage, the tissue that cushions joints, is made up of collagen. By offering the essential building blocks for cartilage preservation, a collagen diet helps joint health by perhaps improving flexibility and lowering stiffness.

Collagen has a role in maintaining the strength and density of bones. By promoting bone mineralization, a sufficient collagen consumption may aid in the prevention of diseases like osteoporosis and osteopenia.

3. Tendon and Ligament Health: Strengthening of Connective Tissue Collagen makes up the majority of ligaments and tendon, both of which are essential for joint function. A diet rich in collagen helps to maintain the integrity and strength of these connective tissues, which may lower the chance of injury and increase mobility in general.

Support for Muscles: The fascia that envelops muscles contains collagen, which gives them structural support. Increased consumption of collagen could aid in improved muscular function and recuperation.

4. Gut Health: Intestinal Lining Integrity: Collagen contributes to the intestinal lining's preservation. This is especially critical for those with diseases like leaky gut syndrome since healthy intestinal lining is essential for immunological and appropriate nutritional absorption.

Support for Digestive System: Glycine, one of the amino acids found in collagen, helps the digestive system by encouraging the formation of enzymes and stomach acid. As a result, nutritional absorption and digestion are optimized.

5. Help with Weight Management: hunger Regulation: By encouraging a sensation of fullness, the protein in meals high in collagen can help control hunger. For those trying to control their weight or support weight loss objectives, this may be helpful.

Preservation of Muscle Mass: Maintaining muscle mass requires consuming enough protein, especially collagen. For both general metabolic health and physical performance, this is essential.

6. Wound Healing and Recovery: Collagen Synthesis in Wounds: Collagen plays a crucial function in tissue regeneration and repair during the wound healing process. A diet high in collagen may help people heal from wounds, surgeries, and injuries more quickly.

Decreased Inflammation: Collagen's anti-inflammatory qualities may help create a more healing-friendly atmosphere. Collagen has the potential to promote a more seamless recuperation process by regulating inflammation.

7. Better Strength and Thickness of Hair and Nails: Collagen helps to maintain the structural elements of hair and nails. A diet high in collagen may result in stronger nails, less brittle hair, and better-looking hair texture.

Brittle nail prevention: By keeping the nail bed healthy, collagen helps minimize the risk of developing disorders like brittle nails.

Including a collagen diet in your diet provides a comprehensive approach to health, supporting the health of important body components in addition to treating cosmetic issues. There are several advantages to eating a diet high in collagen, including joint flexibility and skin regeneration. To optimize these beneficial benefits, it's critical to stress a well-rounded and nutrient-dense strategy that includes a range of collagen sources and supplementary nutrients. To ensure that dietary decisions are tailored to each person's needs and health objectives, always seek the advice of medical specialists or nutrition experts.

HOW TO FOLLOW THIS COLLAGEN DIET

A collagen diet consists of consuming particular meals and choosing foods that encourage the body to produce and maintain collagen. This is a thorough guide that will help you adopt and follow a diet high in collagen:

1. Give Collagen-Rich Foods Top Priority: Bone Broth: Have a filling cup of bone broth to start your day. Bone broth, whether handmade or purchased from a store, is a great way to get minerals, amino acids, and collagen. Think about using it as a stew or soup basis.

Lean Proteins: Make sure your meals contain lean protein sources including fish, poultry, chicken, and lean beef cuts. The necessary amino acids required for collagen formation are provided by these proteins.

2. Include Vibrant Fruits and Vegetables: Vitamin C-Rich Foods: Eat a range of vibrant fruits and vegetables that are high in vitamin C, which is an essential vitamin for the synthesis of collagen. Bell peppers, citrus fruits, strawberries, and kiwis are a few examples.

Dark Leafy Greens: Include Swiss chard, kale, and spinach in your diet. These greens provide vitamins

A and C, which promote the synthesis of collagen and the general health of the skin.

3. Include Nuts and Berries for Antioxidants:

Berries: Rich in antioxidants that fight oxidative stress, blueberries, raspberries, and blackberries are not only delicious but also healthful. Degradation of collagen can be facilitated by oxidative stress.

Nuts and Seeds: Chia seeds, walnuts, and almonds are good sources of zinc and omega-3 fatty acids. Collagen production and skin health are enhanced by zinc and omega-3 fatty acids.

4. Consume Omega-3 Fatty Acids from Fish: Fatty Fish Include fatty fish in your weekly meals, such as mackerel and salmon. Omega-3 fatty acids, which have anti-inflammatory qualities and promote skin health, are abundant in this fish.

5. Pick Sensibly Collagen Supplements:

Collagen Supplements or Powder: If your diet is lacking in certain nutrients, think about including collagen powder or supplements into your regimen.

Supplements containing collagen can be blended into drinks or smoothies.

Select High-Grade Items: To ensure a higher grade of collagen, look for supplements made from animals grown on pasture or grass.

6. Restrict Sugar and Processed Foods:

Cut Back on Sugar Consumption: Reduce the amount of processed sugar you eat since too much sugar can cause glycation, which deteriorates collagen. Choose natural sweeteners sparingly, such as honey or maple syrup.

Steer clear of processed foods: These items are frequently loaded with preservatives and chemicals that can exacerbate inflammation. When possible, choose entire, unprocessed meals.

7. Moderate Alcohol and Caffeine Consumption: Restrict Alcohol Intake: Drinking too much alcohol can cause skin dehydration and disrupt the production of collagen. Drink plenty of water to counterbalance the occasional alcoholic beverage.

Control Your Caffeine Intake: While a modest amount of caffeine is usually fine, too much of it can cause the skin to become dehydrated. Drink water and herbal teas to stay hydrated.

8. Remain Hydrated: Consume Water: For general health and skin suppleness, hydration is essential. Make sure you consume enough water each day to sustain skin cell hydration and collagen's overall efficacy.

9. Examine Cooking Methods:

Techniques for Cooking Rich in Collagen: Include cooking techniques like boiling and slow cooking that maintain the collagen content. These techniques aid in the extraction of collagen from connective tissues and bones.

10. Track the Results of Your Diet:

Note Any Modifications: Observe how your body reacts to the food high in collagen. Track alterations in joint suppleness, skin texture, and general health.

Consult a Professional: For individualized guidance, speak with a medical professional or a qualified dietitian if you have any particular health issues.

In summary, implementing a diet high in collagen necessitates a thoughtful and well-rounded approach to food selection. You may encourage collagen production and advance general health by consuming foods high in collagen, getting antioxidants from dietary sources, and changing your way of living. Keep in mind that every person has different demands, so it's best to speak with medical specialists or nutritionists to customize your collagen diet to meet your unique objectives and take your health into account. The long-term advantages of a food plan that emphasizes collagen will come from consistency and an all-encompassing approach to health.

COMPLICATIONS IF THE RIGHT DIET ISN'T ADOPTED.

Adopting the incorrect diet can have a number of negative effects on the body, particularly when it comes to maintaining collagen health. Inadequate nutritional support can exacerbate the breakdown of these vital structures since collagen is a fundamental protein that is needed for the health of skin, joints, and connective tissue. The following examines the potential issues that might occur from not adhering to the appropriate diet:

1. Skin Aging and Deterioration: Elasticity Loss: Over time, the skin becomes less elastic in the absence of adequate collagen support. This hastens the aging process by causing drooping, wrinkles, and fine lines to appear.

Dryness and Dehydration: Insufficient collagen consumption may result in the skin's inability to retain moisture, which can cause dryness and a dull complexion.

2. Joint Stiffness and Discomfort: Decreased Cartilage Integrity: The protecting tissue between joints, cartilage, is mostly composed of collagen. Reduced cartilage integrity from inadequate collagen support can cause joint stiffness and pain.

Increased Susceptibility to Injuries: Joint stability and the likelihood of injuries can both be harmed by weakening tendons and ligaments.

3. Compromises to Bone Health: Reduced Bone Density: Collagen is essential to the strength and density of bones. Low bone density can be caused by inadequate collagen support, which raises the risk of fractures and diseases like osteoporosis.

Delayed Healing: In the absence of the best collagen support, fractures and bone injuries may take longer to heal.

4. Concerns About the Gut: Leaky Gut Syndrome: One factor that contributes to leaky gut syndrome is a deficiency of collagen support, which can weaken the intestinal lining. Unwanted chemicals can enter

the circulation as a result of this illness, which may cause inflammation and intestinal problems.

Deficiency in the intestinal lining can make it more difficult for vital nutrients to be absorbed, which can have an adverse effect on general health.

5. Problems with Muscle Weakness and Recovery:

Decreased Muscle Support: The fascia that envelops muscles contains collagen, which gives the muscles structural support. Weakness in the muscles and reduced structural integrity can be caused by insufficient collagen.

Extended Recuperation: Insufficient collagen support can cause muscles to heal from injuries or training more slowly, which might affect overall physical performance.

6. Compromised Wound Healing: Delay in Tissue Repair: Collagen plays a critical role in tissue regeneration and repair throughout the wound healing process. Insufficient collagen can cause

wounds to heal more slowly, which raises the possibility of infections and other problems.

Increased Scarring: Larger, more noticeable scars may emerge as a result of inadequate collagen support during wound healing.

7. Compromised Hair and Nail Health: Brittle Nails: The nail bed's ability to retain collagen is crucial. A lack of collagen support can result in brittle nails, which raises the possibility of breaking and other problems with the nails.

Modifications in Hair Texture: Insufficient collagen support can affect the structural integrity of hair, resulting in brittleness, altered texture, and heightened vulnerability to harm.

8. Inflammatory Conditions: Chronic Inflammation Chronic inflammation may be exacerbated by a diet deficient in nutrients that assist collagen formation. Chronic illnesses and autoimmune disorders are among the many medical ailments that are associated with persistent inflammation.

Anguish and Unease: Prolonged inflammation can cause pain and discomfort in many body regions, particularly the joints and muscles.

In conclusion, there are numerous and significant side effects that can result from consuming an improper diet that promotes collagen health. The effects affect many body systems, ranging from accelerated aging and poor skin health to joint stiffness, weakening bones, and decreased gut function. Prioritizing a healthy, collagen-rich diet that includes a range of nutrient-dense foods that promote collagen production and general wellbeing is essential to reducing these problems. Always seek the advice of medical specialists or nutritionists for individualized dietary recommendations based on each person's unique health requirements.

CHAPTER 4

BREAKFAST RECIPES

1. Collagen-Boosting Smoothie Bowl:
Ingredients:

- 1 cup mixed berries (blueberries, strawberries, raspberries)
- 1 banana
- 1/2 cup Greek yogurt
- 1 scoop collagen powder
- 1 tablespoon chia seeds
- 1/4 cup granola

Preparation:

1. Blend mixed berries, banana, Greek yogurt, and collagen powder until smooth.
2. Pour the smoothie into a bowl.
3. Top with chia seeds and granola for added texture and nutrients.

2. Protein-Packed Collagen Pancakes:
Ingredients:

- 1 cup oat flour

- 1 scoop collagen powder
- 1 teaspoon baking powder
- 1/2 cup almond milk
- 1 egg
- 1 tablespoon honey

Preparation:

1. In a bowl, mix oat flour, collagen powder, and baking powder.
2. Add almond milk, egg, and honey, and whisk until well combined.
3. Cook pancakes on a griddle until golden brown on both sides.

3. Avocado and Smoked Salmon Toast with Collagen-Infused Spread:
Ingredients:

- 2 slices whole-grain bread
- 1/2 ripe avocado
- 2 ounces smoked salmon
- Collagen-infused cream cheese
- Fresh dill (for garnish)

Preparation:

- Toast the whole-grain bread slices.
- Mash the ripe avocado and spread it evenly on the toast.
- Top with smoked salmon and a generous layer of collagen-infused cream cheese.
- Garnish with fresh dill.

4. Greek Yogurt Parfait with Collagen Granola:

Ingredients:

- 1 cup Greek yogurt
- 1/2 cup mixed berries
- 1/4 cup collagen granola
- 1 tablespoon honey

Preparation:

1. Layer Greek yogurt in a glass or bowl.
2. Add mixed berries on top.
3. Sprinkle collagen granola over the berries.
4. Drizzle honey for sweetness.

5. Collagen-Infused Chia Seed Pudding:
Ingredients:

- 2 tablespoons chia seeds
- 1 cup almond milk
- 1 scoop collagen powder
- 1/2 teaspoon vanilla extract
- Sliced kiwi and mango (for topping)

Preparation:

1. Mix chia seeds, almond milk, collagen powder, and vanilla extract in a jar.
2. Stir well, cover, and refrigerate overnight.
3. Top with sliced kiwi and mango before serving.

6. Spinach and Feta Omelette with Tomato Salsa:
Ingredients:

- 2 eggs
- Handful of fresh spinach
- 2 tablespoons crumbled feta cheese
- Collagen-rich tomatoes (diced)

- Olive oil for cooking

Preparation:

1. Whisk eggs and pour into a heated, oiled pan.
2. Add fresh spinach and feta on one side of the omelette.
3. Fold the omelette and cook until eggs are set.
4. Top with collagen-rich diced tomatoes and serve.

7. Collagen-Infused Acai Bowl:

Ingredients:

- Acai smoothie pack
- 1/2 banana
- 1/4 cup almond milk
- 1 scoop collagen powder
- Toppings: Granola, sliced strawberries, coconut flakes

Preparation:

1. Blend acai pack, banana, almond milk, and collagen powder until smooth.

2. Pour into a bowl and top with granola, sliced strawberries, and coconut flakes.

8. Quinoa Breakfast Bowl with Collagen-Rich Fruits:
Ingredients:

- 1/2 cup cooked quinoa

- 1 tablespoon almond butter

- Collagen-rich fruits (e.g., kiwi, pineapple, mango)

- Chopped nuts for garnish

Preparation:

1. Mix cooked quinoa with almond butter.

2. Top with collagen-rich fruits and garnish with chopped nuts.

9. Collagen-Boosting Oatmeal:
Ingredients:

- 1/2 cup rolled oats

- 1 cup almond milk

- 1 scoop collagen powder

- 1 tablespoon maple syrup

- Sliced bananas and nuts for topping

Preparation:

- Cook rolled oats in almond milk until creamy.

- Stir in collagen powder and maple syrup.

- Top with sliced bananas and nuts.

10. Coconut and Pineapple Collagen Smoothie:

Ingredients:

- 1 cup coconut water

- 1/2 cup pineapple chunks

- 1 scoop collagen powder

- Handful of spinach

- Ice cubes

Preparation:

1. Blend coconut water, pineapple chunks, collagen powder, spinach, and ice cubes until smooth.

2. Pour into a glass and enjoy this tropical collagen-boosting smoothie.

These breakfast dishes offer a scrumptious and nourishing way to include foods high in collagen in your daily diet, promoting general health and wellbeing. Adapt serving sizes to your dietary requirements and tastes.

CHAPTER 6

LUNCH RECIPES

1. Grilled Salmon Salad with Avocado Dressing:

Ingredients:

- Grilled salmon fillet

- Mixed greens (spinach, arugula, kale)

- Cherry tomatoes, halved

- Cucumber, sliced

- Avocado dressing (avocado, Greek yogurt, lemon juice)

Preparation:

1. Place grilled salmon on a bed of mixed greens.
2. Add cherry tomatoes and cucumber slices.
3. Drizzle with homemade avocado dressing.

2. Quinoa and Chickpea Buddha Bowl:

Ingredients:

- Cooked quinoa

- Chickpeas, roasted with spices

- Sliced carrots and cucumber

- Avocado slices

- Tahini dressing

Preparation:

1. Arrange cooked quinoa in a bowl.

2. Add roasted chickpeas, sliced carrots, cucumber, and avocado.

3. Drizzle with tahini dressing.

3. Collagen-Infused Vegetable Stir-Fry:

Ingredients:

- Tofu or chicken strips

- Broccoli florets

- Bell peppers, sliced

- Snap peas

- Collagen-infused soy sauce

Preparation:

1. Stir-fry tofu or chicken in a pan.

2. Add broccoli, bell peppers, and snap peas.

3. Drizzle with collagen-infused soy sauce.

4. Spinach and Feta Stuffed Chicken Breast:

Ingredients:

- Chicken breast
- Fresh spinach leaves
- Feta cheese, crumbled
- Lemon juice
- Olive oil

Preparation:

1. Butterfly the chicken breast and stuff with fresh spinach and feta.
2. Drizzle with lemon juice and olive oil.
3. Bake until chicken is cooked through.

5. Collagen-Boosting Lentil Soup:

Ingredients:

- Red lentils
- Carrots, diced
- Celery, chopped
- Collagen-rich tomatoes, diced
- Vegetable broth

Preparation:

1. Cook lentils, carrots, celery, and tomatoes in vegetable broth.
2. Simmer until lentils are tender.
3. Season with herbs and spices.

6. Mango and Shrimp Quinoa Bowl:
Ingredients:

- Cooked quinoa
- Grilled shrimp
- Mango chunks
- Avocado slices
- Cilantro-lime dressing

Preparation:

1. Combine quinoa, grilled shrimp, mango, and avocado in a bowl.
2. Drizzle with cilantro-lime dressing.

7. Collagen-Infused Turkey Lettuce Wraps:
Ingredients:

- Ground turkey

- Lettuce leaves

- Shredded carrots

- Collagen-rich bell peppers, sliced

- Hoisin sauce

Preparation:

1. Cook ground turkey in a pan.
2. Assemble lettuce wraps with turkey, shredded carrots, and sliced bell peppers.
3. Drizzle with hoisin sauce.

8. Caprese Salad with Collagen-Rich Balsamic Glaze:

Ingredients:

- Fresh mozzarella, sliced

- Collagen-rich tomatoes, sliced

- Fresh basil leaves

- Balsamic glaze (reduced balsamic vinegar)

Preparation:

1. Arrange mozzarella, tomatoes, and basil on a plate.

2. Drizzle with collagen-rich balsamic glaze.

9. Chickpea and Collagen-Rich Veggie Wrap:
Ingredients:

- Whole-grain wrap
- Chickpeas, mashed
- Collagen-rich vegetables (bell peppers, spinach, tomatoes)
- Hummus spread

Preparation:

1. Spread mashed chickpeas on a whole-grain wrap.
2. Add collagen-rich vegetables and a generous layer of hummus.
3. Roll into a wrap and enjoy.

10. Collagen-Infused Salmon and Asparagus Foil Pack:
Ingredients:

- Salmon fillet
- Asparagus spears

- Lemon slices
- Olive oil
- Garlic, minced

Preparation:

1. Place salmon and asparagus on a sheet of foil.
2. Drizzle with olive oil, add minced garlic, and top with lemon slices.
3. Seal the foil pack and bake until salmon is cooked.

These lunch meals use nutrient-rich items to enhance general health while providing a variety of collagen-boosting alternatives. Adapt ingredients and quantities to suit individual dietary requirements and tastes.

CHAPTER 7

DINNER RECIPES

1. Baked Lemon Herb Chicken:
Ingredients:

- Chicken breasts
- Lemon juice
- Fresh herbs (rosemary, thyme)
- Garlic, minced
- Olive oil

Preparation:

1. Marinate chicken in lemon juice, fresh herbs, minced garlic, and olive oil.
2. Bake until chicken is cooked through and golden brown.

2. Collagen-Infused Vegetable and Quinoa Stir-Fry:
Ingredients:

- Tofu or shrimp
- Mixed vegetables (broccoli, bell peppers, snap peas)

- Cooked quinoa

- Collagen-rich soy sauce

Preparation:

1. Stir-fry tofu or shrimp with mixed vegetables.
2. Add cooked quinoa and drizzle with collagen-rich soy sauce.

3. Salmon and Avocado Salsa:
Ingredients:

- Salmon fillets

- Avocado, diced

- Tomato, diced

- Red onion, finely chopped

- Cilantro, chopped

Preparation:

1. Grill or bake salmon fillets until flaky.
2. Mix diced avocado, tomato, red onion, and cilantro for a fresh salsa topping.

4. Mushroom and Spinach Stuffed Bell Peppers:
Ingredients:

- Bell peppers, halved

- Mushrooms, chopped

- Spinach, chopped

- Quinoa or lean ground turkey

- Tomato sauce

Preparation:

1. Sauté mushrooms, spinach, and quinoa or ground turkey.
2. Stuff bell peppers with the mixture and bake until peppers are tender.
3. Top with tomato sauce before serving.

5. Collagen-Rich Lentil and Sweet Potato Curry:
Ingredients:

- Red lentils

- Sweet potatoes, diced

- Coconut milk

- Collagen-rich tomatoes, diced

- Curry spices (turmeric, cumin, coriander)

Preparation:

1. Cook red lentils and sweet potatoes in coconut milk.
2. Add diced tomatoes and curry spices. Simmer until flavors meld.

6. Grilled Turkey Burgers with Collagen Guacamole:

Ingredients:

- Lean ground turkey
- Whole-grain burger buns
- Collagen-rich avocado, mashed
- Lime juice
- Sliced tomatoes and lettuce

Preparation:

1. Shape ground turkey into patties and grill until cooked.
2. Mix mashed avocado with lime juice to create collagen guacamole.

3. Serve turkey burgers on whole-grain buns with guacamole, tomato, and lettuce.

7. Vegetarian Collagen-Boosting Stir-Fried Tofu Noodles:

Ingredients:

- Tofu, cubed
- Vegetable noodles (zucchini or sweet potato)
- Collagen-infused stir-fry sauce
- Sesame oil
- Green onions, sliced

Preparation:

1. Sauté tofu until golden.
2. Add vegetable noodles and stir in collagen-infused stir-fry sauce.
3. Drizzle with sesame oil and top with sliced green onions.

8. Cauliflower Rice and Shrimp Bowl:
Ingredients:

- Cauliflower rice

- Shrimp, peeled and deveined

- Collagen-rich vegetables (bell peppers, peas)

- Low-sodium soy sauce

Preparation:

1. Sauté shrimp and collagen-rich vegetables.
2. Add cauliflower rice and stir in low-sodium soy sauce.

9. Collagen-Infused Chicken and Vegetable Skewers:
Ingredients:

- Chicken breast, cubed

- Cherry tomatoes

- Zucchini, sliced

- Red onion, wedges

- Olive oil and herbs for marinating

Preparation:

1. Marinate chicken cubes and vegetables in olive oil and herbs.

2. Skewer and grill until chicken is cooked and vegetables are tender.

10. Spaghetti Squash with Collagen Pesto:
Ingredients:

- Spaghetti squash
- Grilled chicken strips
- Collagen-rich pesto (basil, pine nuts, collagen powder)
- Cherry tomatoes, halved

Preparation:

1. Roast spaghetti squash until strands can be pulled.
2. Toss with grilled chicken, collagen-rich pesto, and cherry tomatoes.

These supper dishes provide a range of collagen-rich choices to help you meet your nutritional requirements. Depending on dietary restrictions and personal tastes, change the ingredients and serving sizes

CONCLUSION

To sum up, adopting a collagen condition diet is more than just a matter of what foods to eat; it's a dedication to nourishing the basic components of our bodies. The collagen-rich diet shows promise as a comprehensive strategy for general well-being, promoting bone density, gut health, and skin renewal in addition to joint flexibility.

The wide variety of recipes—which include breakfast, lunch, and dinner—offers a gastronomic adventure that satisfies palates while providing vital nutrients for the synthesis of collagen. Including foods such as salmon, berries, leafy greens, and collagen supplements gives you the essential vitamins, minerals, and amino acids that keep your skin, joints, and connective tissues structurally intact.

Always keep in mind that consistency is essential when you start this revolutionary diet. Conscious, little decisions add up over time to provide long-term advantages. Beyond the obvious benefits, the collagen condition diet is an opportunity to cultivate a more intimate relationship with your body by recognizing the mutually reinforcing relationship between your dietary choices and your overall well-being.

Thus, let this change in diet become more than just a habit; let it symbolize your dedication to wellbeing and vigor. Imagine the strong bones, flexible joints, and tough skin your body is creating as you relish each collagen-rich meal. Allow the mirror to reflect not just your outward beauty but also the radiant wellness that emanates from inside.

Consider your body as a painting and the collagen condition diet as your palette as you embark on your path to overall well-being. Each nutrient-dense morsel adds to a work of health and energy art. Accept this gastronomic journey as a celebration of your body's amazing ability to flourish rather than as a limitation. The collagen condition diet is more than simply a decision; it's a self-gift that demonstrates the fundamental relationship between nourishing yourself and thriving vitality. Enjoy the tastes, bask in the advantages, and use the collagen condition diet as a blank canvas to create a colorful, prosperous life. This symphony of wellbeing is your body's due, and you are the conductor crafting its beautiful tune.

Contact Us

Dear Reader,

If you have any questions, need further clarification, or require assistance with any aspect of the book, please do not hesitate to reach out to me. I am more than happy to provide additional insights, address your queries, or simply engage in a meaningful discussion.

Feel free to contact me at: IsabelleHartleyBooks@gmail.com. Your feedback and inquiries are always welcome.

FREE 30 DAYS MEAL PLANNER

FREE 30Days Meal Planner, a priceless extra to get you started on the path to a more organized and healthy living. This meticulously curated planner is made to make meal planning easier, save you time, and help you meet your nutritional objectives. Prepare to enjoy the advantages of this wonderful resource! Scan the QR Code below now.